Mammograms, Mastectomies, and
Mom's Apple Pie:

My Recipe for Handling Breast Cancer
and
Returning to a Healthy Life

Vickie Jenkins

Mammograms, Mastectomies, and Mom's Apple Pie: My Recipe for Handling Breast Cancer and Returning to a Healthy Life

Copyright © 2011 by Vickie Jenkins

Cover Design: Carlo Carmona

Cover Illustration: ©Margarets/Bigstock.com

Interior Illustration: ©iStockphoto.com/hfng

Back Cover Photo: Todd Brown

ISBN 978-1466451421

"It's Breast Cancer Awareness month."

My friend Carlo looks up from his laptop at Priscilla's Gourmet Coffee Shop. "You gonna write it?"

I sigh. "Yeah. I guess I'm ready now."

Yesterday in follow-up treatment at the clinic, the nurses sat me between two brand-new chemo patients. One squeezed her eyes shut during the entire two hours, and barely breathed. The other talked excitedly in Spanish to her husband, who held her hand and translated. I opened conversation with each of them, giving them tips the doctors and nurses don't know, because they're just watching, not living it. I was old hat now, eight months in.

Last month a friend whose mom was diagnosed with cancer asked me to write down what I had done to recover, so I began to chronicle what had happened with my own treatment and the things I learned and applied to help me.

This book is not about what treatment to choose. It's not a technical report. It's not about the history of the disease. I figured there were plenty of cancer books out there that covered all that.

This book is simply a series of successful actions—both traditional and non-traditional—that I took to speed up my recovery from breast cancer surgery and chemotherapy. And the bizarre, ironic, comedic moments that accompany the harsh reality of handling a body crisis.

I always had the goal of – "Handle it, and get back to health."

If that is also your goal, perhaps some of the tips in this book might help you. Or you can at least have a laugh or two at the sillier stories.

But in the end you design your own program. Your health is your responsibility and it all begins with the attitude you take.

Survive? Or Succumb.

I write this book in my birthday month—October—which is also Breast Cancer Awareness Month here in the U.S.—of which I am much more aware now.

I am celebrating another birthday, another year on this planet. I give thanks to all who helped me—family, friends, medical specialists, spiritual leaders, and fellow explorers.

I dedicate this book to YOU, the readers—and to the next worlds that you will create as a healthy, glowing spirit.

Much Love,

VJ

Table of Contents

PART 1

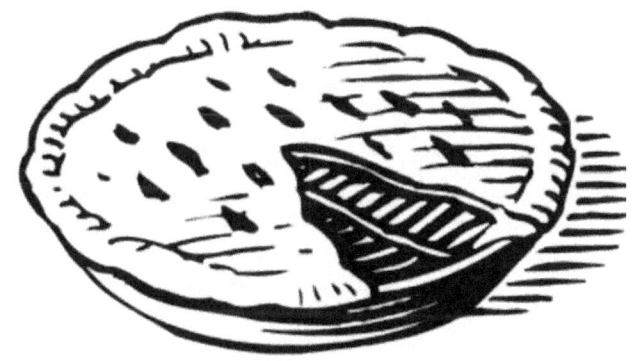

1.

Not I, Said the Frog: The Lump

"Lots of people have lumpy breasts."
"I barely have breasts—let alone lumps."

I found it while lying in bed one March morning.

I was home sick with the whatever-you-get-when-a-nasty-person-lands-on-your-communication-lines-and-you-don't-recognize-it illness.

A small, hard lump on my right breast. Smaller than a marble. Kind of.

I was barely working as a consultant during the recession, and had no health insurance. Well, there was nothing I was going to do about it, I decided.

That was a mistake.

Looking back, I recall a line from the story of the Little Red Hen, about HELP—helping others and helping yourself:

"Who will build the fire?"

"Not I," said the frog.

2.

Okay, Here's the Deal: The Confront

Definition of confront: (verb) to face without flinching or avoiding.

"I gotta tell you something."

I looked into my doctor's bright blue eyes.

"There's a lump on my right breast."

"Well, let's do a full check-up then."

I took off my blouse and put on the gown, laid down on the examination table.

He felt around both breasts, carefully, with a female nurse present.

When I was dressed he said, "You need to get that checked. Now."
This doctor was a fairly quiet-voice type, but this time I detected a sense of urgency.

He wrote up the lab order for the sonogram and mammogram.

"Get these tests done now. This week."

Seemed a bit of a rush, since I'd now had the lump for at least eight months, but—okay.

I called the lab, with two obstacles—they had no openings for three weeks and the cost was prohibitive.

For years I had been an employee, always with health insurance, seldom using it. Now I wasn't and I needed it and didn't have it. So I checked around and found a program that offered free mammograms where they could fit me in the next week.

Here we go.

"There's the second one."

"The second what?"

"Lump."

I was lying on the table with my arms up, the cold gel sliding the sono-gram probe around my right breast, when the technician stopped it dead in its tracks as I watched the monitor over her shoulder.

I'd only seen sonograms used to find fetuses—healthy heartbeats, teeny toes, shifting shadows. This picture looked like a black mass. Next to another black mass. Two lumps.

My mind flashed to a joke, as it often does in crisis.

"Sugar? One lump or two?"

Two, next to each other.

I heard the same urgency in the voice of the doctor who came in later to read the images. "We'll need to do a needle biopsy—as soon as possible." That turned out to be the following week.

The Breast Center is as nice a place as you can build, considering the people and equipment there are designed to diagnose and treat trouble.

Female patients sat in muted-tone chairs, gowns wrapped tightly around them, waiting their turn, thumbing through magazines loaded with pictures of perfect women with perfect smiles in perfect bodies. Every one of 'em had two boobs. Some may have been implanted, but they had 'em.

The waiting women hung their heads, silent. Not a smile among them.

As I waited in the mammogram room next to giant, shiny equipment that would soon be pinching my breasts—again—I selected specific things in the room to look at, to help me stay calm and in present time.

I kept it up until my breathing was steady and I was able to confront things in the room without freaking out.

I used to get freaked out easily—something my former therapist called an "anxiety attack" — but hadn't a clue what to do about it. I left that 'treatment' behind and actually learned a way to handle those moments—without drugs, without side effects—bringing me back into present time, and smiling.

After the technician took multiple pictures of both breasts with the mammogram machine, we moved back to the sonogram room, where I got shots in the right breast to numb it, and then I watched the computer screen as they guided a needle into each dark spot in the breast to snip out pieces to send to the lab.

The sonogram technician and two doctors were extremely nice to me during the procedure, making small talk to distract me from the snip and suck process. When it was finished they all smiled at me. But I saw the flicker of concern in their faces. *They already know. They've done this a thousand times and they already know.*

By the way—as part of this 'core needle biopsy' they take chunks out, then mark the inside of your breast by implanting tiny metal pieces in different shapes for each lump, to mark where they've taken samples. I got a tiny knot and a ribbon embedded in my right breast. So—would I set off alarms at the airport body scanners? No, they said. Shucks. That would have been exciting.

All this happened after Thanksgiving. By Christmas I was looking at the small bruises and stitches on my right breast and apologizing to it for putting it through so much trauma.

Christmas week I waited for the results. And waited. And waited. My doctors were on holiday. I wasn't.

Finally the biopsy results were faxed to my doctor who called to have me come in ASAP. I hate that phrase.

3.

Betty Was Right: The Diagnosis

First, You Cry.

I kept remembering that book title from fellow newswoman Betty Rollin, and boy, did she nail it.

I sat there in the extra room they have at the end of the hall at my doctor's office. The one where you sit and react after you're received the bad news. Just before you get your shit together and start planning your treatment.

But first, you cry.

My doctor was straight forward with me. She's done a lot of spiritual work as well as medical treatment, and she told me that with Stage III breast cancer there is no 'drink grape juice' or 'seaweed treatment' or alternative programs out there that had successful survival statistics. "At Stage III, those people are not around anymore."

I got it.

So, let's proceed with the standard medical treatment, which has worked successfully on 100,000 women just like me. Go directly from A to B without a circuitous route thru Q, Z, Y or anything else, and get this handled.   ASAP.   Now I liked that phrase, I decided.   And the DECISION to act is everything.

I wasn't giving up the spiritual work. But I was adding to it, with full-force medical treatment.

Within a week I was at County Hospital, filling out forms, meeting with specialists at the breast clinic, and setting dates. Los Angeles County even has the Breast and Cervical Cancer Treatment Program, which helps pay for surgery and follow-up medical care for women who have no medical coverage.

The doctors said I could either have a lumpectomy (cut out a part of the breast where the lumps were) then do radiation and chemotherapy, or have a mastectomy (take off the entire breast) skip radiation and do chemo. I figured, "What am I gonna do with half a breast?" and if that helped me avoid radiation—great. So I voted for the mastectomy plan, then it had to go to the Tumor Board for review and approval. The Tumor Board. Can you imagine how much fun THOSE weekly meetings are? They approved my plan. We set the surgery date.

I exhaled, for the first time in about a week.

4.

Family Prayers, Friendly Action: The Plan

"You've moved to the top of the family prayer list."

My sister, on the phone from Home. I laugh, and tell her "Well, I knew I'd be Number 1 back there someday."

Home is a small farm town in the middle of corn country, with a Main street that once thrived, now on its last legs, displaced by Wal-Mart and a faster-moving world. A place where I could still walk down the street years after being gone and someone would stop me and say, "Hey, aren't you one of the Jenkins girls?"

The town population there is the size of one of the high schools here in Los Angeles, home to 9 million strangers. You'd think I'd feel alone here, far from family, but I'd long since collected my own family of friends, and with the help of my own church group, I was facing this body issue with a plan and support.

So I didn't tell my family back Home until after the mastectomy. It had been scheduled for, coincidentally, my sister's birthday, so I didn't call her until a few days later. I wanted to make sure my plan was in place so I could keep myself and others calm as we worked it through and prepared for post-surgery cancer treatment.

And I had to figure out how to say it.

My sis took it well, as did all of my brothers and sisters, sending love and support and prayers. Soon we were having regular phone conversations, emails, and cards and letters about it.

Each person makes his or her own decision about who to tell and when, based upon your relationships and your attitude about how you will handle the condition and how others will react.

I found it was best to keep people around me who focused on the plan, the positive attitude, and the future—not getting bogged down in "poor you" or re-telling stories of everyone they've ever known with that disease. Here was my favorite: "My friend had breast cancer surgery and got through just fine. 'Course she drank herself to death later on, but…"

PART 2

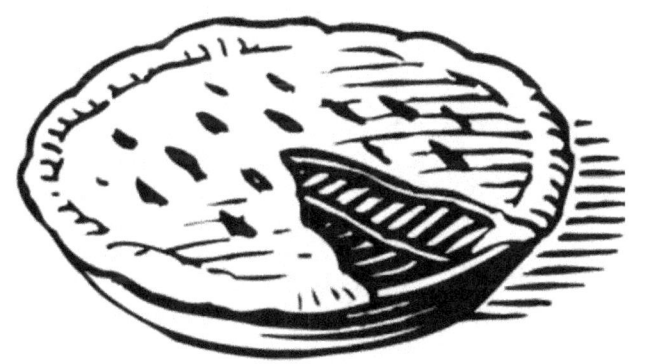

5.

Is That a Recipe Book?: The Surgery Prep

So, how do you prepare for surgery? Well, you get your body and your environment in order.

That means double-checking all of your medical paperwork and medicines, paying all your bills ahead of time, selecting what to take and wear to the hospital, making sure you have lots of high-quality vitamins (tablets or liquid), buying food since you won't want to cook when you get home, and laying out the house in a quiet, simple manner so that it's easy for you to get around—slowly—while you recover.

So even though it's before surgery, you're preparing for after surgery.

Always think in futures. Moving ahead, planning recovery.

I meet with friends, lots of hugs and smiles. Just a couple of tears. I have 'action' friends. So when I tell them what's happening they say, "Okay. Got it. What's the plan?" And they're on board. But they let me remain at cause—not effect, not telling me what to do, but asking me what else I need, and offering suggestions.

That distinction is rather important. When you are the effect of something, you are not in control. You go to the doctor who uses a bunch of big words and you hear "cancer" and you blank out and you're in a strange environment full of mystery and unknowns so you slide further and further down into apathy, letting others run the show, because you don't have enough information to make any decisions on your own.

But if you study and ask questions and learn about the treatment and your active part in it, you can remain much more at cause and heal more quickly. That is KEY.

So I asked a lot of questions and made notes about what the surgery would entail, what I should bring and not bring to the hospital, how and where my friends should be during the surgery, when I would be discharged, etc.

The surgery was a mystery no more. Okay.

Oh—the title of this chapter. Yeah.

As part of being cause instead of effect over life, I knew I would need to stay positive and keep my thoughts directed as I waited for the operation. So I took my little spiral book of spiritual study with me to the hospital room and as I sat there in my gown waiting for the attendant to come get me for surgery I was reading and highlighting the book that discussed our abilities as spiritual beings, how big and powerful we are when we realize it.

The doctor came in, looked at the spiral-bound book, and asked "Is that a recipe book?"

I smiled. "Yeah. Kind of."

When he left I looked at the woman in the next bed. She was two days out of surgery and suffering. Since she spoke only Spanish and I did not, I needed another way to communicate with her.

I knew she too was a strong, powerful spirit. I could see it. I sent her the thought—"You'll be alright."

I simply smiled at her and nodded. She smiled back.

Translation not needed.

6.

Did You Eat?: The Surgery

That light is out.

My thought as I am wheeled into the elevator on a bed, laying there looking up at the fluorescent tube under the plastic ceiling light cover. It's a totally different view, seeing the world only in ceilings.

The attendant navigates the bed into the room next to the surgery room and tells me the doctor will be right with me.

I look at the clock on the wall. Surgery is three hours late. It's now almost 3:30 and I know the doctor and her team has been in the operating room handling bodies since 7 a.m.

When she arrives and comes to my side, she asks, "You haven't eaten right?" to make sure that I won't get sick while under anesthesia and start throwing up, which can be quite dangerous. "No, not since last night" I tell her. "But did you and your team eat?" I ask. She smiles. "Yes."

You know how sharp you are when you're tired and hungry, right? I don't want the people with the scalpels and drugs in that condition. Okay good. The team is ready. And so am I. I put my smile and trust in her and her team. I know we will be fine. Now I leave the work up to the doctors.

They move me to the operating room, open up my arms wide and strap them down to boards on either side of me, so that when they cut off the cancerous breast and take nodes from the lymph glands under my arm, I won't move. I'm laying there like Jesus on the cross. Jesus.

The anesthesiologist smiles at me as another team member slips the breathing apparatus over my nose and mouth. "Good night Miss Jenkins."

Note: Everything that is said by anyone in the operating room while you are under anesthesia is recorded in your mind. It's true. Your mind keeps recording everything during every moment of your life, even when you're unconscious. You can actually recall it later when you're wide awake. In case you want to know what the team said or did while you were sleeping.

7.

Let's Get Out of Here: Post-surgery Recovery

"Nodes negative."
The doctor whispers to me as I come up out of the post-surgical fog. I smile. *Cool. So the cancer did not spread from the breast to the lymph nodes under my arm. Upward and onward.*

I go back to sleep.

Post-surgery is a bizarre environment. The nurses wake you up every 90 minutes throughout the night to see if you need any drugs to help you sleep. Or if you need more drugs to handle your pain. Well if I was in pain, I probably wouldn't be asleep. I have one nurse's assistant who is so sleepy herself that she starts to take my blood pressure on the surgical arm, which you're never supposed to do. I stop her in time and she realizes what she's doing, and switches to the other arm.

Holy Moses. You gotta keep your eyes open even when you're asleep.

After that I sleep with one eye open. Except when they slip me drugs to sleep, while I'm asleep. Like I said, the mind records EVERYTHING. *I see you.*

The next morning another doctor (*holy mackerel he's cute*) comes in to change my chest bandage and check my vitals. Everything looks good. "Are you in any pain?" he asks. I'm numb from my neck to my waist.

"No" I answer.

By noon I'm starving and finally ready to take in some food. I sit up—slowly, get dressed—slowly, and dig into a delivered turkey dinner with dressing, green beans, milk and strawberry shortcake dessert that's to die for. Who says hospital food is awful? This tastes like a feast after 36 hours on empty.

Note to friends of surgery patients: If you call the room to see how we're doing and we don't answer—don't panic. We're probably knocked out. Call back later and just ask the nurse to check on us, because there's a good chance we can't even complete a sentence yet, let alone carry on a phone conversation. This is serious dope we're getting in the hospital.

As a matter of fact, when I'm dressed and ready to check out, another nurse comes by.

"Do you want something to go?"

"What do you mean?" I ask, "Like, iced tea, or—"

"No. Pain medication," she says.

Yikes. Drugs to go. I mean, a drive-in Starbucks is one thing, but…

"Uh, no, I'm good," I answer. "Thanks anyway."

"Well if you want it—I just have to watch you ingest it before you leave."

"No really, I'm okay."

By the time my friend Sue arrives at 1 p.m. to pick me up and take me home, I'm roaming the halls, moving at the speed of mud. She's surprised I'm not in a wheelchair, head hung low. But I have the spiritual tools and the help of friends. And no drugs to go.

"Let's get out of here" I tell her. "This place is full of sick people."

I know we've got healing to do.

8.

The Secret Weapon: Body Communication

"I'm gonna move that toe!"

I have no idea how old I was when I first watched John Wayne and Dan Dailey in the 1957 John Ford-directed movie *The Wings of Eagles*, but I clearly remember the scene and that phrase.

Wayne played the lead in the real-life story of a Navy pilot whose accident left him paralyzed from the waist down. In the movie, his buddy Dailey would come in every day and say or sing or shout to get him to repeat the phrase, "I'm gonna move that toe!" Wayne would lay there face-down on the bed, staring into the mirror so he could see his toes. Day after day, week after week, they worked together until Wayne was able to move one toe, then a foot, then a leg.

When you've suffered some type of body trauma, the body shuts down, and needs help waking up. So the more time you spend getting back in communication with it, the better off you are.

We never want to touch something that hurts. But you need to let all those body parts know that it's gonna be okay now.

My friend Sue was my Dan Dailey, helping me become more able to confront the body.

When my toes were numb I'd touch them and say, "Hi there. Come back, come back, it's okay now. Come on." Then we'd do the same thing with my shoulder, my arm, my chest. Touching and connecting all those body parts.

She and I actually started this body communication work BEFORE the breast surgery, and continued through post-surgery and chemo.

Sometimes when we'd do the work, I would yawn and feel dopey, pushing through all of that anesthesia and drugs to get back into communication. And my body would heal. And heal. And heal.

So besides doing the traditional physical therapy to get my surgical arm moving again with that big scar across my chest, I was also getting help using a non-traditional approach, to prepare me for chemotherapy one month after surgery.

Family, friends, and doctors were amazed at how quickly I recovered and how well I looked, despite the trauma.

Anytime you have a physical pain, burn, etc., try communicating with that body part. And buddy up with others to help them do the same.

No matter where we are on the healing curve, we can all get better, can't we?

PART 3

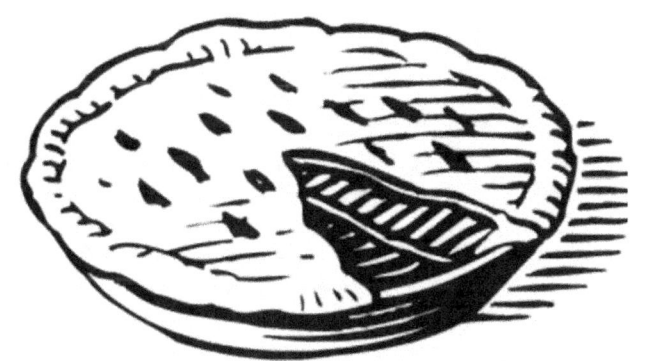

9.

Red Bells, Yellow Bells: Not Just 'Physical' Therapy

Speaking of getting better—
Stay with someone when you get home from surgery.
You're as weak as a new-born baby, and about as self-sufficient.

In a later section of this book I go into details of how to set up the house to make it easy after your operation.

In the first few days at home after breast surgery, I was numb numb numb. And dopey dopey dopey.

My exercise consisted of walking around Carlo's apartment or down the hall and yawning a lot. Eating chicken broth or soup. And sleeping and sleeping and sleeping. Figuring out a position to sleep in without being in serious pain. Which side of the bed to sleep on to easily roll out and get to the bathroom. Waiting for Sue to arrive after work to help me. And sleeping and sleeping and sleeping.

It's also a good idea to have strong-stomached friends around to help you take the surgical wrap off of your chest. You don't want to confront that flat chest and big scar alone. Here's how mine went:

Carlo: "Okay, you ready?"

I nod yes.
Carlo cuts the bandage off, slowly unwraps it.
I look down.
I start to cry.

Carlo: "What are you doing? Is that crying? There's no crying in cancer!"

He's paraphrasing Tom Hanks from the movie *A League of Their Own* and I burst out laughing. The tears stop.

About those red bells—
In surgery the doctors put a drainage system in your chest, to make sure the lymph nodes fluid and chest fluids don't build up in the weeks after your operation. Which means you wear drainage bags.

They're called the Jackson Pratt drain, or JP drain. No one seems to know who invented them at Jackson-Pratt, but the predecessor—the Penrose drain, was invented by Charles Bingham Penrose in the late 1800s before they had silicone or plastics, and consisted of surrounding the gauze bag with an ordinary rubber condom with the end cut open. Penrose, by the way, was a wild man—who survived a bear attack, swam 15 miles through the ocean on a dare, overcame tuberculosis, and escaped a lynch mob in Wyoming. (Sorry. This is what happens when you spend too much time Googling a topic on the Internet.)

Anyway—back to the Jackson-Pratt drain. The drainage tubes stay in your chest and they're connected to the outside of your body to a pair of collection bulbs that you empty twice a day. You tape them to your waist or use safety pins to attach them to your pants or shirt. Some people think they look like hand grenades. Okay, not my favorite visual when I'm recovering from cancer surgery. They actually look like bells, once you empty them.

You squeeze the fluid out of the plastic/rubber bulb into a measured paper cup, then push the bulb back together so it makes a bell-shape. As the fluid fills up the see-through bell, you can see the fluid—red or yellow, or almost clear. Your goal is less fluid emptied each day (you keep daily stats) until eventually you have empty bells.

After surgery you also do physical therapy exercises to regain use of your 'surgical arm'—the one that had lymph nodes taken out of it and the side where your breast was removed. They may cut out a piece of your chest muscles as well as the breast, so moving the arm is a slow process, as you re-build your arm strength and are able to move it higher and higher.

When I'm well enough to shuffle one block down the street (accompanied by Sue) I look at the outside world and begin to feel the space around me open up again. Fresh air. Flowers. A far-off mountain. Space. Oh, there I am. Bigger than the body. I'm a big spirit. Aaaaah.

I buy over-sized long shirts at the thrift store to hide my red and yellow bells when I go out. I can handle the way they look, but someone standing next to me at the grocery store looking down and asking themselves, "Is that BLOOD in that thing?" might pass out. Hide the bells. Please.

I wore the red and yellow bells for two weeks, and then the technician pulled them out. In one big yank. Yikes.

If you're interested, I have pictures of the entire process—from diagnosis through surgery to chemo, baldness and re-building. I take pictures of everything—a lovely sunset, a delicious plate of food, a chest with incisions.

As soon as you're well enough from the surgery, they start you on chemotherapy. For me, that was one month after the operation.

I thought I'd been through the roughest part. Silly me.

10.

Agua, Por Favor: Chemo Prep

"Did your husband get his chemo treatment booklet—in Spanish?"

"The only one they had in our language was for ovarian cancer."

That's a real conversation I had with some poor soul at the hospital.

Particularly when you're heading into chemotherapy, there's a lot of stuff you need to know and get ready for, so make sure you get the proper information—written information. Preferably in your own language.

READ IT. And any word you don't understand, stop and look up the definition and use it in enough example sentences until you really know the meaning of that word. If you don't, and you just breeze past that misunderstood word, all the information after that will be a blank in your mind.

At one point I had an oncologist who kept slipping into "medicalese" during our conversations while I was trying to take notes. I'd put up my hand and say, "Hold it! What does that mean?" As patients we can only do our part if we understand what the heck is going on. So look up the words or ask the medical staff to explain, in plain language.

That written material, plus your regular appointments with the doctors and nurses, will really help you prepare for chemotherapy—explaining the treatment, your medications, side effects, warning signs, medical test schedules, and your diet.

Chemotherapy takes hours and hours. It's not like taking your car in for an oil change. Trust me on this one.

So—to prep for chemo, put together a travel bag of everything you need to keep you occupied for six to eight hours. That might be a book, a video, music, or beautiful peaceful pictures. One woman did her crocheting, although I couldn't figure out how she managed it with the I.V. stuck in her hand.

Bring food. I never felt sick until about 48 hours after chemo, so I needed plenty of food while I was hooked up during treatment. If you get hungry you get kinda crazy, and you don't need any stimulation for that in this environment.

To prep for chemo one of the most important things to remember is DRINK WATER. You need to flush your system before, during and after the chemo is pumped into your body.

As a matter of fact, the chemo poisons are so nasty, that the directions say that in the first 48 hours after chemo you're supposed to flush the toilet TWICE every time you go to the bathroom.

So—mucho aqua, por favor. Not Pepsi, Red Bull or coffee. Aqua. Mucho mucho aqua.

Gracias.

11.

Fully Armed: Chemo, Shots, Drugs

Did I mention aqua, por favor? I brought a six-pack of waters from the 99-Cent Store every time I went in for chemo. Keep drinking, keep peeing. Yes, you have to unplug your chemo machine from the wall and let it run on batteries while you roll your bags of meds hooked up to your arm with you into to the bathroom to urinate, but trust me, you learn how to navigate that move. Just remember to plug the machine back in when you return to your chair or bed.

Keep drinking. Keep peeing. And double-flush. Por favor.

Chemotherapy takes HOURS. You've got the paperwork, check-in, blood tests, vital signs (blood pressure, heart rate, temperature) and weigh-in, then needle insertion into a vein where they will be pumping the chemo into your blood stream, pre-meds (medication you take before the chemo), saline fluid, and then the famous brown bags—the actual chemo chemicals—in specially-marked brown bags and handled with heavy-duty gloves because they're so nasty, checked and double-checked before they're hooked up and pumped into your veins. My typical time for the entire chemo cycle was check-in around 10 a.m., wrap up around 5 p.m. Or 6.

Here's the deal. If you DON'T bring something to do, you sit there and stare off into space and your reactive mind takes over and you can get kinda crazy. That's why the nurse asks you, "Do you want something to stay calm?" Personally I figure I'm on plenty of drugs and don't want another one that messes with the brain. So to keep calm on your own, bring things to do to keep you occupied.

Some people bring a loved one, but carting the entire family into the treatment center for "support" is unacceptable. Those nurses have work to do and they can't be navigating around snoring Uncle Harry, your weeping mother saying the rosary over you in three languages (just to make sure) and your nieces and nephews who are playing video games and yakking on their cell phones.

Give your fellow chemo-ites (I just made that up) a break. Leave the family drama at home. We're tryin' to heal here.

You also have a long laundry list of drugs to coordinate during chemo. Drugs to take the day before, during and after. Drugs to take if you feel nauseous. Drugs to keep you from having rashes. Drugs to help you move your bowels. Take this one three times a day, take two of those twice a day but only the day before, take that one if you feel sick but not more than once every 12 hours, take this on an empty stomach, never take that on an empty stomach…

It's a lot. Keep a list. Get others to help you keep track. Because let's face it, you're doped up. And you're expected to drive home from chemo. Seriously.

As part of my chemotherapy I had to learn to give myself shots. After each chemo your white blood cell count drops and the shots of medicine are designed to help your bone marrow make more white blood cells. Of course you get weird pangs of pain in your bones when the bone marrow stimulation drug kicks in, but hey, that's just another fun side effect of chemo.

That means you have to learn to give yourself a shot. With a needle. No closing your eyes and turning away while someone else does it.

This is another level of confront.

But they've got these cool "how-to" videos for you to watch over and over until you learn how to do it. Do it exactly as they say and you'll be fine.

Here's the weird part for me. I come from an entire family of diabetics. Everybody but me has diabetes. I have cancer. Go figure. Anyway, I've watched family members give themselves shots for years. Shots in the arm, the leg, the stomach. But ME give MYSELF a SHOT? Heck no.

Well, it's heck yes.

Sue or Carlo would help me set up each time, making sure I had the alcohol, medication, needle, syringe, cotton balls, and band-aid all laid out in a sanitized place. Then I'd do it step by step, just like the video said, with my support standing by. I was so scared, my legs would shake.

After each shot we had a celebration, and a count-down of how many more shots I would have to give myself during the treatment cycle. I had five days of shots after each chemo treatment. One day I'd give myself a shot in the left leg. Next day, the right leg. Then the left side of the stomach. Next day the right side. Hey if my brothers and sisters could do this…

Step by step. Keep moving forward.

On the final shot day—there were 30 of them in all—Sue and I grinned and cheered. Score! Another win.

Celebrate every win, kids. Really.

12.

Farting at the Library: Handling Side Effects

It was one of those awful squealers.

I was at the Amelia Earhart Public Library in North Hollywood, California. A great old mission-style Spanish building from 1929, re-named for the female aviator who disappeared over the Pacific in 1937.

At this moment I wanted to disappear.

The fart sounded like the air you slowly let out of a balloon when you squeeze and pull the neck of it. High-pitched. Lasting forever.

But—you feel these things coming on and can suppress them, right?

Not in chemo.

They show up out of the blue—while sitting, walking, laying in bed.

They're not stinky, just—noisy.

And in the silence of that soft-filtered sunlit room of the library, this one was thunderous.

But as it squealed out, no one looked up. No one would look at the bald girl.

Go ahead. I dare you. Don't make me take off this hat.

Actually I was grateful nobody looked. Because my netbook was not big enough for me to hide behind.

Later, telling a friend, we had to laugh about it. I mean, what else can you do? You're bald, with scabs on your face, looking like you crawled out of a tomb, and now your chemo-filled beat-up body is making weird noises in public. Great.

Now, amid this vision of Vickie the farting bald girl, I will share with you some of the possible side effects of chemotherapy, all of which I experienced:

> Bone pain, red dry spots on hands, sores in mouth, throat, and on face, skin shedding, itchy sores around the vagina and anus, swollen neck glands, infections under the skin near veins, itchy red spots on neck, itchy palms, chest pressure, heart palpitations, shortness of breath, acid reflux, nausea, constipation, hair loss everywhere (I mean EVERYWHERE), swollen legs, foot, ankle and leg cramps, swollen red face, nosebleeds, runny nose, intestinal cramps, gas pains, numb tongue, numb toes, purple toes, toe pain, brittle nails, headache, fatigue. And— FARTING.

You can imagine how much fun I was to be around. From one end of my body to the other end, I was dripping, oozing or squealing, with fast fierce pains in between.

But when I wasn't cussing I was laughing. As each new painful or weird side effect hit me, I would yell, "Somebody shoot me!" But luckily my friends ignored that.

Besides keeping track of the drugs and side effects, you have to identify how to handle specific body problems that come up:

If you have a fever, CALL THE DOCTOR.
If something looks or feels like an infection, CALL THE DOCTOR.
If you get chest pains and they feel serious, CALL THE DOCTOR.

If you're farting—GO HIDE IN THE CLOSET.

Some side effects are just a pain. When my ankles disappeared and were replaced by two legs that looked like tree trunks, I asked the doctor about the fluid retention. He said I could take one of the pills I was on the day before each chemo. "But isn't that a corticosteroid?" I asked. He paused. (I'd been doing my online drug research). "Uh, yeah. But it only causes swelling if you take it for 30 days or more."

I knew this was not true based upon MY EXPERIENCE. The first day I took that little pill my face got round and full and red.

So I went back online to find foods that worked as natural diuretics, that is, foods that would help me release water or fluid from the body. I made the list of foods and bought them and ate them: watermelon, asparagus, and cranberry juice, among others. I peed and peed and within 24 hours my ankles were back to normal.

As my sister says about always following the doctor's advice: "It's still YOUR body."

Today I'm reminded of that. In the trial of Michael Jackson's death, one of his employees said when they asked Michael about all the drugs he was taking he said "My doctor says I have to, so I do." We lost an incredible creative soul. But his music lives on with us. My two favorites: "Man in the Mirror" and "You Are Not Alone" which I play to keep my spirits up.

At the height of chemotherapy when there was a battle going on for my body—between the drugs and the cancer—I was so exhausted, angry and sick that I cried and fought. I thought, "Really, I can't do this anymore." But I would hear that reactive mind statement and make a new choice — survive or succumb? *Not yet, bud. Get outta here, negative thought.*

Then I'd do something about it, such as read my spiritual books or listen to music or watch a favorite movie or—hell, just take a pill and sleep. I'd close my eyes and run the calendar in my mind.

Four more treatments, VJ. Then you're through. Or—three more sets of shots, VJ. That's 15 more. You're half-way through. Keep going.

My family and friends would do the same—mark their calendars, follow my stats and keep me going, with comments, cards, encouragement. Every step, every small cycle of action completed, was a win.

Be strong. Be strong.

I toyed with getting a yellow wristband, but I'm not really into jewelry. And besides, I didn't plan on keeping this cancer or its memory anyway.

As a loving famous man once said, "Upward and onward."

I agree, sir. I agree.

PART 4

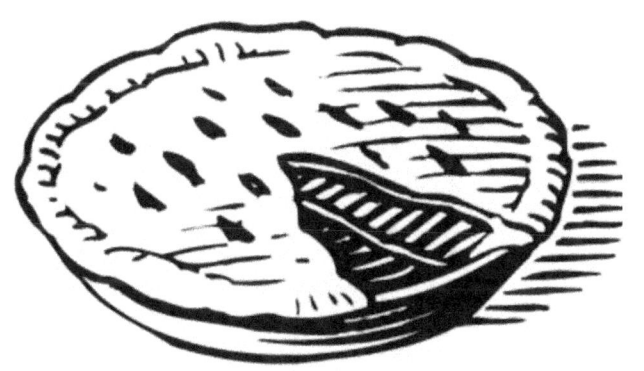

13.

Life Imitates Life: Giving and Receiving

At Oncology Clinic today I see the tiny buds sticking out of a plastic cup of water. I recognize them. They're daffodils, not yet showing their color, but soon. Daffodil Days is the annual fund-raiser for the American Cancer Society, which I supported when I was on-air at KOIT Radio in San Francisco.

Daffodils are the first sign of spring, the first signal that life is re-emerging after a long, hard winter. I have old pictures of me delivering daffodil bouquets to breast cancer patients at the hospital. Me, standing there with long black hair—them, bald or in turbans.

The irony of my past and present does not escape me.

When I was in radio news in San Francisco I had many connections to this disease. I emceed walks, runs, and golf tournaments—for breast cancer.

I interviewed survivors, researchers, and charity workers—for breast cancer.

I even won a national award for my series on breast cancer awareness, flying to Washington D.C. to accept the honor from CBS's Leslie Stahl.

Now, I was on the receiving end.

So I can attest to how your donated money is used.

The various programs, including Look Good, Feel Better, Revlon/UCLA Breast Center, Avon Cares for Life, the American Cancer Society, and Cancer Care helped me get tests and surgery, a wig when my hair fell out, makeup to brighten up my pale face, a fake boob insert to a special bra when they cut off my breast, and gasoline to get me back and forth to weekly blood tests, emergency room visits, oncology appointments, and chemotherapy.

Please support me in the Cycle for Breast Cancer program.

"Will do, Larry," I write back in his email. "But I'm handling it myself right now." He'll pedal faster.

Come walk with my team in the fight against breast cancer.

"Would love to, Rosie, but I'm in chemo right now," I answer online. She says her prayers are with me, but she knows me from our years together in the news biz in San Francisco, and tells me she isn't worried.

"Would you like to donate to a cure for breast cancer?" the grocery store clerk asks me this week, at the start of Breast Cancer Awareness Month.

"Sure."

Because it helps people.

14.

Great Haircut!: Cancer Camouflage with Wigs, Boobs, Makeup

"Great haircut!" the woman at the pool-side cocktail party says to me.

"Thanks!" I smile.

It's working. The cancer camouflage is working.

I'm halfway through chemo, bald, slightly scabby, and bloated, but none of it shows tonight at this publishing industry event I attend to keep my toe in the business.

Here's what I used from the various cancer programs:

Wig. I got to pick the color and the style, a short, cute blonde-brown mix. I've also bought colorful scarves as head wraps, and I have more fun hats now than I've ever owned. They even gave me a headband with just bangs hanging from it that you can wear under a cap, so it looks like you've got hair! Cool.

Boob. I'm in Hollywood, so I could have gotten falsies anywhere, but as part of the hospital program, I am fitted for a fake boob and special bra. I try on different sizes, weights and shapes of boobs, complete with nipple. They all feel so HEAVY to me. But that apparently was the weight of my breast plus muscles, now gone. The new boob bra feels good and with a built-in camisole piece across the center, I can even bend over and no one can see down my shirt to the flat-chested scar. After breast surgery, when you look down your shirt, you don't see cleavage, you see the floor.

"I never thought I'd end up selling boobs," the prosthesis specialist tells me. "Well, you help a lot of women, and I thank you for that," I respond. She is positive and happy, because I know she knows she is helping.

PS: Yes I know I could have gotten reconstructive surgery to build a new breast but I have no interest in any more operations. Besides, this way I can also wear my old bra and stash my money, car keys, and Kleenex in the empty right-side cup.

Makeup. The American Cancer Society has a "Look Good, Feel Better" program to help you keep a healthy-looking face while in treatment, and after the group makeup session you get to keep the cosmetics you've applied.

Larger Clothes. I've bought new thrift store pants 2 sizes larger, since I'm GAINING weight on chemo. This is unfair. I mean, I lost a pound or two by taking off the right breast. But since I take pills to stop throwing up in chemo, I keep my food down and my weight up. And I retain fluid from all the chemicals and drugs in my system. I've gained 10 pounds on chemo. "Make sure you're eating," my sister tells me. *Please. I'm dying for an Astroburger and onion rings right now. I'm eating I'm eating.*

By trying all these new looks and adapting them as the body changed, at some point in treatment I just let go of what people thought of me and my body. I decided I could be anyone I wanted, not just the old me.

I could be a Hollywood hipster—with a bald head, full makeup, big hoop earrings, and a painter's cap.

I could be a gypsy-pirate, in a colorful head-wrap, baggy white blouse gathered under a wide black belt, and black pants.

I could be a corporate communicator, in a wig, business suit, makeup, and tiny pearl earrings.

I was just dressing up the body and playing parts. And even though some of my parts were missing, I simply replaced them.

As a matter of fact, one evening I looked up in the bathroom mirror and my bathrobe had slipped open. *Holy mackerel! There's a part missing! A boob!* And I laughed and laughed. Then I went into the bedroom and began to take artistic pictures—of the baldness, the body, in shadows and angles. It was a work of art. It was nothing to be ashamed of or sorry for.

I don't remember dressing up as a kid. I was a tomboy on the farm, making mud pies, playing with the animals, not caring how I looked.

Later, I began to agree with the universe that said I "should" be this or I "should" act that way.

Not anymore.

It was also at this point that I began to write again, a talent which I had shut down for a couple of years. I resumed writing poetry. I revived and am finishing my murder-mystery novels set in 1950s L.A. I pulled out my comedy screenplays to sell. And I began making notes of funny things in my environment.

My girlfriend Suzy had given me a 'healing diary' before my surgery, encouraging me to write down any thoughts, poems, or reflections. And so I have.

The cancer camouflage actually gave me the chance to un-cover ME.

But that was just the beginning of the joy.

15.

Cancer-Free. What a Lovely Phrase: Returning to Life

"Well, since you're cancer-free you can…"

"What?"

The oncologist had said it so quickly that it almost slipped past me.

"You're cancer-free. We got it all at the site. And now the chemo has covered the rest of the body. All we have left to do is the Herceptin therapy every three weeks, for a year."

I'm still on the phrase "cancer-free."

I somehow knew it, but to hear the doctor say it out loud meant that I could also repeat it to others.

And I did.

Whenever someone would come up to me, hug me, and ask, "How's it going?" I could now say, "I'm cancer-free!"

They were soooooooo excited! It is a win for everyone.

So now I am in the therapy that blocks the cells from receiving future signals about growth, and that is also delivered into my veins every three weeks using the man-made protein Herceptin. The side effects involve the heart and lungs, the blood circulation. But so far my heart is tolerating it pretty well, and they check it every few weeks with an echocardiogram.

Of course, after walking up one flight of stairs, I'm pretty much done for the day. But that's nothing compared to what I've been through. I'm not oozing and itching, paining and shedding.

As a matter of fact, my hair's coming back. My head looks like that of a baby chick, newborn out of the shell.

I AM a new chick!

I let people feel my fuzzy head (might as well help them confront cancer as well) and they smile. "Oooooh. It's soft." Yes. Everybody likes newborn chicks.

I ask them if they have any questions about this cancer or my treatment. I don't want others to be in mystery or fear about it, and I'm comfortable discussing it.

And when I go to the hospital every three weeks now, I can help others who are just starting chemotherapy. Back in the beginning I couldn't even look at the bald-headed patients. Now I'm one of them, and I smile and wave. We are a brotherhood of survivors.

I tell one of my sisters that I'm writing a book about my experience with breast cancer and how I got through it.

"You mean kinda like a 'my life behind bars' story?" she asks.

I laugh.

"Uh, yeah. Kinda."

I know that we are here to help each other, and to be free. And to stay on the positive track.

Which isn't always easy when the universe keeps trying to convince us this is all we've got.

But I'm no longer listening to that.

Are <u>you</u>?

16.

What are YOU Looking At?: The Healthy Info Diet

"Please join us in the auditorium for today's Department of Medicine lecture – Infectious Diseases."

Why are the pictures, conversations, and focus at a medical facility constantly reminding us of disease?

I go to Cardiology to get an echocardiogram to see how my heart is holding up during chemo. At the window there's a 3-D plastic life-sized form of an open heart with a clogged artery that every patient gets to look at when they arrive. It's sponsored by a drug company, I see on the corner of the display. Ah-hah! Thanks for reminding me, just in case I forgot and instead had a thought and future vision of what a HEALTHY HEART MIGHT LOOK LIKE.

In Oncology there are giant pictures of cancer cells.

In another clinic, there's a diagram on the wall of a really sick colon.

If this is medical education, who educates us on how to get well?

We learn by gathering information on our own, experimenting, talking to people. Making decisions and choices on what to eat, do, say, think, and treat.

I couldn't really tell you what to eat when you're going through cancer treatment. I got some crazy cravings myself, and followed them. The important thing was for me to drink lots of water, and to keep my energy up by eating.

"Are you eating?" "Like a Hoover vacuum, Sis. Knock it off."

The American Cancer Society puts out a very helpful booklet called "Nutrition for the Person with Cancer during Treatment." It lists different types of food to eat based upon whether you're in chemotherapy or in radiation, and whether you've got low counts of red blood cells, white blood cells, or something else. Specific problem, specific food. And the book has lots of tips about how to keep your environment clean and sterile to prevent infection. The National Cancer Institute also has a good publication called "Chemotherapy and You." So that's covered.

I'm more concerned about your Information Diet during treatment.

It was best for me to keep my communication lines clean. For example, I would never watch the news. It's a long list of fires, rapes and robberies—and a puppy story at the end. Not such a good balance. You think I'm kidding. Make a list next time you watch.

One day while watching the local news at my sister's house, they literally led with a story about a fire, then a rape, then a robbery at a bank…sorry, I turned it off before they got to a positive story, if there was any at all. If you feel you need to know what's happening, just read a few headlines online. But remember, overall, the news is negative, negative, negative.

It's the same with <u>people</u> around you during treatment. Keep the negatives away from you, by phone, email and in-person. I don't care if they're you're best friend (what kind of friend is that?) or your twin brother or your boss or your mother. If they make you sick, turn them off. You're already sick and trying to get better.

The worst person will be the one who smiles as if helping you, but throws in hidden negative comments that in some way make you feel less than you are. They're smiling as they're sticking the knife in your back. GET RID OF THEM.

You have so much to handle during the treatment of cancer that you need all the positive tools, people, and information you can find. Without overload.

One day, when I was finally able to get out and walk around the block after surgery, I stood under a positively gorgeous flowering bougainvillea tree. There I was, completely surrounded by nature's beauty—living and growing. I took a picture of those flowers on my cell phone and looked at them often over the next weeks and months, sending it to my friends and posting it on Facebook.

As I said, the lists at the end of this book are successful actions I took. Maybe they'll spark some ideas for you to come up with your own solutions. Just include in your healthy diet the things that are:

POSITIVE...POSITIVE...POSITIVE.
NOT NEGATIVE...NEGATIVE...NEGATIVE.

Pictures, movies, music. Things which are so aesthetic, so beautiful, that they lift your spirit up, up, up. Because the higher your emotional tone level is, the faster you can heal.

PS: I dare you to go online and find pictures of <u>healthy</u> cells, and to print them out and look at them daily. Because those are what YOU have to manufacture in your body. The dudes in the white coats and stethoscopes have a different job—to treat the disease. Yours is to create a new, healthy body.

I will create new cells.

And quit lookin' at that sick colon.

PART 5

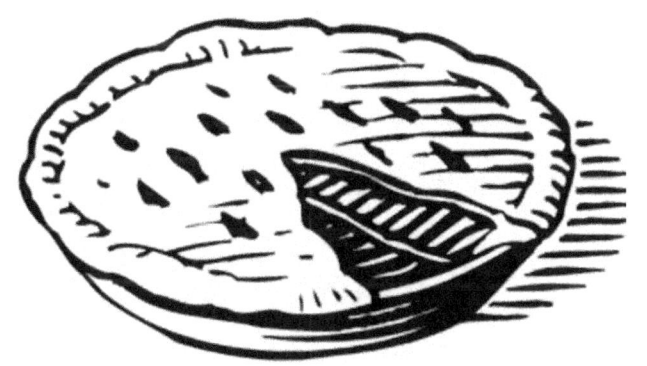

17.

Happiness Re-defined: Abilities Gained

I never really took the time to figure out what 'happiness' meant in my life.

I knew when I wasn't happy. And as I observed strangers on the street I saw that they seldom looked happy.

So, what WAS happiness, anyway?

Well, let's see, shall we?

When am I the happiest?
While sitting on a park bench watching the sunset? Sort of.
Lying in bed on a rainy morning? Eh.
Laughing with friends at a movie? For awhile.
Consuming a delicious meal? Close.

How about when I've won?

Yeah baby.

It doesn't have to be a BIG win. Just a win, that comes after effort.

Have you ever completed a course and gotten a certificate?
Wrapped a team project at work and received a standing ovation for it?
Cleaned the back yard and planted flowers?
Scored a goal just before the buzzer sounded?
Cooked a new, untried meal that turned out great as you toasted with friends?
Or whipped breast cancer's butt, despite multiple obstacles along the way?

That feeling—that ABILITY—is Happiness.

Overcoming obstacles and reaching a goal.

After I was diagnosed, I set about creating my desired goal—to be cancer-free.

Now, as for the obstacles—I had to know them to overcome them. So I had to get out of that mystery world of 'unknown obstacles'—what is this disease and what are the treatments and what are the drugs and how do I handle it and what are the things to ask and…

I was gathering info so I would get out of mystery so that I could identify each obstacle, take action on it, and overcome it—to reach my goal.

Isn't that what you do every time you face a problem? Take it apart piece by piece, gather more knowledge so you can make decisions, then take action, step-by-step, to solve it.

That could be any problem—from software you installed that's not working, to a relationship break-up, to bankruptcy.

I think that's why people, when they retire, if they DON'T have other games to play or other obstacles to overcome toward new goals—they loose interest in life.

Look at TV and film writer/producer/director Garry Marshall. When I talked to him recently at a coffee shop here in Hollywood, he was busy editing his latest film, then his book was coming out, then he was going to return to television. When I saw science fiction/fantasy writer Ray Bradbury, his assistant rolled him into the bookstore in a wheelchair, but he was in games with new goals, overcoming obstacles, talking about his story that was being shot as a film in Japan, and a new book that was coming out, and…

Had they overcome obstacles in their lives? Heck yes. Were they vibrant and active and happy and interested in people, at any age? YES.

Okay. I get it. Happiness. Action.

I set up my schedule—listing the dates for the surgery, then the chemo treatments, and after overcoming each obstacle I would feel like—*yeah!* Keeping my eye on the big goal at the end.

There were setbacks along the way, of course. But as I faced them, with the help of family and friends, each win was a win for all.

You CAN overcome obstacles, reach your goals and know happiness. It is being done by regular folks like you and me every day, in action, all around the world.

And as I read in a birthday card years ago:

Keep moving, or they'll throw a sheet over you.

Hee hee.

18.

The Cancer Discount: Help is a Two-way Street

"You're in AARP, right?"

The manager at Denny's Restaurant says to me, his fingers poised over the cash register.

"What? Uh, no I'm not 55—yet." I answer.

"You're in AARP, right?" He repeats, nodding yes as he says it.

"Uh—yes?"

"Good!" He rings up my bill. 20% off.

Later that day I tell Carlo about it.

"You got the cancer discount."

"The what?"

"Look at you."

I turn to the mirror. Bald head under a pink hat. Pale face. No eyelashes. Drawn-on eyebrows.

"Oh."

People interact with you differently when you have cancer. Or they CAN interact with you differently, depending upon how YOU act.

I look directly at total strangers now, and smile. I grant them beingness, meaning I see them as a true spiritual being, no matter what the body looks like—tall, short, white, black, young, old, biker, preacher, home-less, bejeweled. People enjoy talking to me and I enjoy listening to them. I'm not afraid of them and they tell me all sorts of hopes, dreams and secrets, relieved of the burden.

I get help and give help freely. Because now that I no longer believe, watch or read the daily news, and instead get out and actually interact with people, I find from my own first-hand experience that **man is basically good.**

And I am amazingly happy, having overcome obstacles to reach healthy goals.

Sometimes, when some obstacle looks like Mt. Everest, I think:
I kicked cancer's butt. I can kick this too. Just take it apart, VJ, piece by piece.

So I wrote this book, overcoming a new obstacle (*write a book??!!*) toward my new desired goal: to help you, your family and your friends live a healthier, happier life. I hope.

As I write this, it is my birthday—October 5th. My family and friends are calling with lots of love for a true birthday celebration—I'm here another year! Yippee!! I am so grateful, and ready to give back.

In the middle of the celebration, I get word that we've lost another creative, amazing spirit to body cancer.

Apple Computer Co-founder Steve Jobs gave us, not just the incredible communication tools of Apple, but also Pixar Animation, so I ended my day watching "Cars 2", that colorful, funny movie with a message—about how even when people are making fun of you and how different you are, that you must stay strong and be true to yourself and your friends. Mater may be a rusty old tow-truck, but he is there to help, and he changes people's lives in a positive way, just by being himself.

I know I'm here to help in the largest way I can, without fear, without judgment.

God knows I've long since stopped worrying about the body, confronting everything from scars and baldness to sores and sickness.

At the beginning of treatment when Carlo helped me shave my head I looked like Sinead O'Connor. Then I resembled a holocaust survivor with sores and scabs all over me as the chemo went after every living cell. Then when ALL of my hair fell out I resembled a pre-cog from the movie "Minority Report." And as my hair started to come back, fuzzy and white for some reason, I looked like a giant Q-Tip. When my toenails turned purple from the chemo treatment I bought purple flip-flops to match. I mean really—you gotta roll with it.

Because after all, it's just a *body*. It's not ME. I'm just using it to get along in this particular life cycle.

It's an amazing thing. Your ability to confront and to help others increases with cancer.

And you don't have to shave your legs or dye your hair for months.

19.

Have Your Pie and Eat it Too: Doing What You Love

There are certain smells I love.

Fresh-cut hay.
The earth, after it rains.
Fresh-baked apple pie.

Since I can't always create a harvest, or a rainstorm—
I bake a pie.

It's my comfort zone, something I know how to do well, and I enjoy it.

As a matter of fact, I'm invited to barbecues because of my pie. "Vickie, you're bringing the apple pies, right?" *Yes. Pies. Plural.*

When I move to a new place, I un-pack and bake a pie.
When a friend needs help, I call and then I bake a pie.
When I feel like I don't have control over much (like breast cancer), I bake a pie.

I bring this up because at times during treatment, you may feel like you can't even tie your shoes right.

Just do what you love. And what you do well.

It may be reading a story to a child, or winning at a video game, or making a great cup of coffee or fresh-fruit smoothie.

Or baking a pie.

There's something you're good at, and doing that small thing gives you an immediate win, in the face of a snowstorm called cancer.

Mine is called "Mom's Apple Pie" because—well—my Mom always made it when I was growing up on the farm.

I'd give you the secret recipe, but then I'd have to kill you.

Actually, I just don't measure anything when I cook, which drives my friend Suzy crazy. My Mom's Apple Pie involves plenty of cinnamon, a dash of nutmeg, a pinch of salt, and brown sugar. How much? No clue.

But this is part of my healing recipe: Bake your own pie.

PS: I buy my roll-out dough from the store, I don't make it. I'm not *that* talented.

20.

Prom Night: Celebrating Success

I look at the calendar.

July 8th.

The final chemo treatment.

In the ten days following that event, every side effect re-surfaces to kick my butt, like the climactic ending to Tchaikovsky's 1812 Overture.

Finally, the bombardment ceases.

Whew.

Now my friend Sue and I plan our own version of Prom Night.

I have been living in sweat pants and flip-flops for months, Sue in black business suits. It's time to break out and celebrate the end of the biggest part of breast cancer treatment.

Our church is having its annual Gala in early August, and we vow that I will be healthy enough for us to dress up and party.

We shop for gowns.

Let's go BIG.

Sue finds a super deal on a silver lavendery floor-length gown with layers of ruffles, with matching pink and lavender bejeweled earrings. I pick a bronzy-orange floor-length gown of taffeta and sequins that matches my brown/blonde wig, with gold and sparkly hoop earrings. My gown can be worn with straps or strapless.

Go BIG.

I decide to go strapless. Hey, just because I lost a breast, I am no less a woman.

Besides. This is Hollywood. We can create any illusion we want.

With help from the saleslady at June's in Burbank, we get the false boob into a strapless bra, and with some last-minute sewing, and a LOT of two-sided tape, the dress looks fabulous.

On 'Prom Night' we put on our gowns, makeup, jewelry and high heels (and my wig) and we head out the door.

The church building is decorated like a magic castle, in blues and greens and twinkling white lights. So elegant.

We get our pictures taken on the red carpet. The food, entertainment, entire evening is magical. We celebrate the church's good work and wins helping people around the world, and Sue and I recognize our own wins on the home front.

My friends who have gathered from around the globe—from Colombia, Italy, Venezuela, Sweden, and across the U.S. from Portland to Long Island—don't even recognize me in my magic gown, but when they do, they squeal with delight and hug me. They all look so beautiful in their own gowns, so handsome in their tuxedoes.

At the end of the night we gather around the white piano in the lobby as my friend Eric plays and one of the Broadway stars give us an impromptu concert. Our hearts soar as they create the most amazing music—voices and instrument in perfect harmony.

Back home, out of our pumpkin carriage (also known as Patti Prius, my hybrid car), we change clothes and sleep like babies, filled with joy and gratitude.

You WILL make it to the end of treatment, my friend.

And when you do—GO BIG.

PART 6

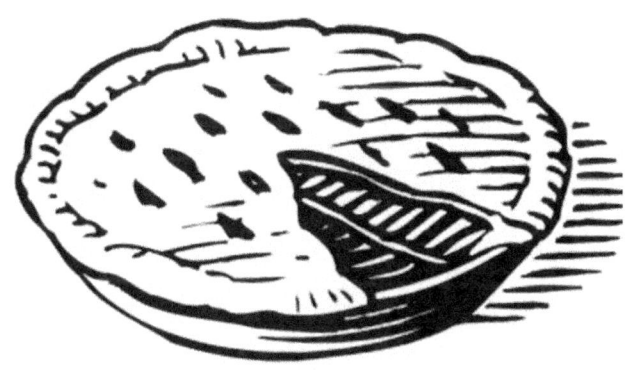

Remembering Me, Remembering You

I am not this body
Or the hair on the floor.

I'm not this scar
Or the headache

I am not this biz card
Or car
Or house
I am anything but

I am a free-flowing spirit
Whipping through the wind
Sliding on Saturn
Shining through the night.

Limitless. Eternal.

You can't see me
Only know me
For as I remember
So do you.

Come out, come out
Come play with me
And realize
You're limitless too.

For we are simply soulful friends
Sharing a laugh and a smile.

But I am not this body.
I just stole it for awhile.

Things I Thought: Mirror Images

Definition of 'to handle': To finish off, complete, end cycle on. I like that.

I'm on the job. I'm here to help.

We'll start an all-girls band of breast cancer survivors. We can call the group 36/0, 24, 36.

Ow! What the hell was that?

Ow! That's right, get in there and kill those cancer cells!

Ow! I'll never make fun of those red-butt orangutans at the zoo again.

Ow! Somebody shoot me.

Chemo – the new Brazilian wax!

No chinny chin chin hair!

I have lost some weight. A pound or two in my chest.

Half-way through chemo! Yeah baby!! Three down, three to go.

Who ordered this body by Grinch? Don't stand sideways in front of the mirror, VJ.

I'm a new chick!

I look like Sinead O'Connor.

I look like a holocaust survivor.

I look like a pre-cog from *Minority Report*.

I look like a Q-tip.

I look like Mr. Clean, minus the muscles and one boob.

Who the hell is that?

I look like— Oh. Hi! It's me. Hee hee.

Take Two Pages & Call Me in the Morning

As with any health crisis, the more organized you are ahead of time the easier it will be for others to help you when you're too sick to handle it all.

The following section breaks down what I did before, during, after, and in between breast cancer treatments. They are only actions that I took, but they were successful actions for me and some may help you as well.

As always, check with your doctors first.

Ask questions. Make notes. Do your research. Build your healing team, including both medical specialists and positive supportive family and friends.

When someone sees me and asks I simply tell people I am "Handling the body," not "I have cancer." I'm not ignoring it, I'm just looking forward.

People will offer their own alternative treatments. Just thank them and continue with your own decision of treatment.

Infection? Hit it FAST. If you have red swelling and/or a fever, call the doctor.

Find something funny or ironic? Write it down! Take a picture, watch a video or movie, write poetry, look at beautiful flowers. Create beauty and laughter and surround yourself with other people who do the same.

My friend Carlo signs his emails with a boxing phrase about persistence: "Six times down, seven times up." Well, with six chemo treatments, that's my new motto too. I may get knocked out each time, but I'm getting back up after every one of them.

Celebrate the small stuff. On Mother's Day I went to a Target store and bought a new purse. I'm not a mother, but who cares? I can still shop the deals, right? When my hair fell out I bought a lovely purple/black striped scarf with sequins.

YOU'LL MAKE IT. AND – YOU MATTER.

My friends get teary-eyed and look at me with such admiration. I am a strong role model for them. Remember that. What YOU do helps others too.

I'm sending you wonderful thoughts!

Much Love,
Vickie Jenkins
Email: vjenkins09@gmail.com

VJs Successful Actions

A: Tips – Before, During, After and Between Treatments

B: Organization – Medical Info, Paperwork, Finances, the Home

C: Shopping List

D: Treatment Journal

A: Tips

BEFORE TREATMENT

Organize your paperwork, household, people, and supplies.

Do all of your shopping before chemo or surgery – get all food, water, videos, music, and supplies (see my Shopping List below).

Get a good night's sleep.

Eat a good meal (if food is allowed before treatment).

Take your vitamins.

Let people know what's happening. Before certain treatments or surgery, I emailed or called family and friends to remind them that I was going in and I would be out of contact for 4-6 days after treatment. I needed to keep quiet and sleep until I felt better—which sometimes took several days.

DURING CHEMO TREATMENT DAY / SURGERY DAY / DOCTOR'S VISIT

Carry a bag of things to keep you busy during the 5-6 hours of chemo or pre-surgery, or a long doctor's visit. Bring a nice book to read, music to listen to, or a project to work on. Bring food, snacks and water.

Dress in layers because the treatment room may be colder or hotter than it was outside the building. If your head gets cold, put on a stocking cap or a scarf with the stocking cap under it.

Talk to other people in the room. Don't just sit inside your thoughts. Help others.

Set your mental thought – "I will come through this just fine."

AFTER SURGERY / TREATMENT

Have encouraging people around after the surgery. Gentle but positive people.

Re-emerge from sleep on a gradient scale, step by step. Get back out into the world. Walk a little bit. Bad weather? Walk in the house hallway. Yawn off all of those drugs.

*Specific Doctor Tip:

My doctor advised me to wait 2-3 days after chemo to start bone marrow injections/shots so I was more recovered from the initial chemo hit.

BETWEEN TREATMENTS

Monitor the body. Fever, Infection? CALL THE DOCTOR.

Get positive uplifting input – funny movies, beautiful pictures & music.

Don't sit around and talk about cancer all the time. Talk about your future plans, and ask what others are doing.

Take walks. Look at things far and near, see beauty. Take pictures of life.

Communicate with your body. Don't be afraid to touch it.

Get out among other living things. Visit a dog park, or a children's playground. Be around LIFE.

If you feel like creating, CREATE. Write, draw, play music. Getting dressed and selecting your look is your creation. Making a meal is your creation.

Help someone else. After surgery I participated in Read Across America Day, reading Dr. Seuss books to second graders. It was so fun and uplifting, and totally got my mind off of the surgery, working with kids who had such great energy. One little girl, who was celebrating her birthday, brought me a donut after the event and told me I was 'the coolest.'

What better healing gift could I have than that?

B. ORGANIZATION

MEDICAL INFO TO CARRY WITH YOU WHEN MEETING WITH HEALTH SPECIALISTS:

_____ Paperwork

_____ Insurance card

_____ I.D. card

_____ Medications

_____ Treatment Journal

_____ Contact names, addresses, phone numbers, email

Communicate with your doctors. Do not let them use words that you don't understand! Stop the doctor and ask, "What is that? In common language." Make them speak slowly and clearly enough so that you can TAKE NOTES. Repeat it back so you understand it correctly. Or you can record the conversation and play it later to transcribe.

Do NOT let them print out something that's so technical you'll get lost reading the first line.

Double-check everything – drugs, dates, times, paperwork, test results. Workers make mistakes. LOOK at nurses, doctors, and administrative personnel. Are they there or are they on 'automatic pilot'? Engage them in conversation to make sure they are THERE. Hello? Anybody home?

Make navigating the medical system a game. Drop off your prescription refill while waiting for the blood test, or the doctor. Find ways to beat the slow-moving system.

MEDICAL RESEARCH / EDUCATION

Everyone has an opinion of what you should do. "Go to Venezuela" "drink grape juice." "There's a greens program." "Heat therapy." Thank them, take in what is right for you, and make your own decision.

Once you have selected your treatment, go do it, and focus on the goal–health.

I found the traditional "support groups" were sometimes too sympathy-based and focused on illness, not health. They were stuck in their illness, telling and re-telling stories.

Double-check information at multiple websites to make sure it is accurate.

Limit your Internet time. Don't focus all your time on research, drugs, problems. Go watch a cat video and laugh.

PAPERWORK

Get organized. Make a medical treatment file to store papers.

Ask for copies of reports and prescriptions.

Read everything you get from the doctors and other health specialists. Watch the "how to" videos.

Keep a treatment journal. Note the date, time of treatment, weight, blood pressure, pulse, blood tests, discussion, follow-up action, etc.

Select your team of 'Navigators' to help you get through the system. If your hospital does not have specialists who coordinate your treatment schedules and financial paperwork, ask an efficient friend to be your personal 'Navigator.'

Set goals, stay busy.

This is a marathon, not a sprint. One step at a time.

FINANCIAL ASSISTANCE

Medical bills can be overwhelming.

As soon as you are diagnosed, contact your employer, credit card companies and other creditors to let them know of your medical condition and hardship. Hopefully they will work with you. If not, consider having an approved consumer credit counseling service negotiate payments for you, or check out filing for bankruptcy. I used an excellent book from Nolo Press, listed in the websites/references section of this book.

When I contacted one credit card company and told them I was moving in with friends to help me handle breast cancer, their customer service person replied, "So you have a new address for us to send the bills to?" I asked them about lower payments and she said, "We used to do that but not anymore. I'd like to help you but the computer won't let me."

Groups for you to contact for help:

Government Programs (state, local, and federal)

Hospital / Physician Groups

Employer

Credit Counseling / Financial Management Agencies

Charities to help you pay for food, gasoline, wigs, a prosthesis: American Cancer Society (or the equivalent in your community), Cancer Care and others.

HOUSEHOLD

Keep the house clean and quiet.

Stay away from pets (scratches or insect bites get infected!) and other germ carriers, which may include kids or anyone who has a cold/illness.

If you have no one to wash the dishes, use paper and plastic ones. You won't feel like cleaning or doing dishes.

Keep clean – use lots of hand soap, paper towels, toilet paper, garbage bags, and pure olive oil to keep your skin soft after washing.

Always have KLEENEX tissues nearby! Your nose will run either with mucus or sometimes blood.

Keep an extra waste basket near your bed in case you get sick. Put plastic bag liners in waste baskets to make them easy to empty. Since you're using a lot of paper towels and Kleenex, expect to fill them up often.

Use a large hand-held mirror – so you can see what's happening on all parts of your body.

Have soft uplifting music nearby.

Only watch TV programs that are light, funny, or positive. Nothing heavy or noisy or negative.

Read/watch/listen to uplifting spiritual information.

Keep the "sympathy" "poor you" and "grief" people away. You need positives only! Your recovery depends upon you staying up-tone, with up-tone support from others.

Save money during treatment by shopping at the 99-Cent Store, Target, and thrift stores. You will be using a lot of paper products to stay clean and sanitary, so shop for deals. Oh, but all that paper and plastic and waste is bad for the environment. I know. GET OVER IT. We're trying to survive cancer.

FOOD

Buy food the day before chemo and have everything at home already prepared for 3-5 days—chicken soup, etc.

Pick the foods that work for you. Check the cancer treatment nutrition books.

Vitamins – I used multi-vitamin packets and replaced the B vitamin with a 'no niacin' B vitamin because I didn't want a 'flush.'

Drink lots of water every day, to clean out your system. Not colas or caffeine. If you get bored with water, mix in apple or cranberry juice.

BODY

Prep – cut your hair. (I said goodbye to my hair stylist, for awhile). When you start to shed like an angora cat, it makes less mess in the house and the shower drain if you just cut off your hair.

You might lose weight but prepare to gain weight as the body retains water with all the chemicals.

Clean the area after each urination. Use unscented baby wipes and Vagisil or a generic brand to handle the sores/itching in the vaginal area. The nurses said to flush twice every time I use the toilet in the first 48 hours after chemo—that's how poisonous the stuff is! That's why I started cleaning the area with baby wipes immediately after every urination. Get those chemicals off the skin!

Wash your hands often and use paper towels. Do NOT re-use hand towels (germs).

Keep your hands and face soft with olive oil.

Do NOT shave with a razor. You may cut yourself – bleeding is hard to stop. Use an electric shaver.

Use nail clippers and a nail file to keep your fingernails and toenails short so you won't accidentally scratch yourself while sleeping. Infections happen so easily when your white blood cell count is low.

Later in chemo your fingernails may get very brittle and split. Take gelatin and use fingernail polish to protect them from catching on things and tearing off.

Plan to look good – fake boobs, hats, scarves, wigs, fake bangs, or au naturel.

Share pictures with positive friends – "Look- here's my new wig/hat/buzz cut."

TEETH

Use a soft toothbrush, and brush with baking soda in water. No toothpaste or mouthwash. It stings and has alcohol.

Gargle and rinse your mouth with warm salt water to prevent mouth sores.

Do NOT floss teeth. Causes bleeding. If gums bleed, rinse with warm salt water.

GASTRO-INTESTINAL

Sleep sitting up to prevent stomach acid back up.

Take Prilosec or Zantac over-the-counter drugs to prevent acid reflux. Also, keep extra-strength chewable TUMS nearby.

For short-term aches and pains the doctor had me take Advil—but not aspirin or any blood thinner.

Take a bowel loosener to keep your system moving. You have to eliminate the toxins with urination and bowel movements. Magnesium works (such as in the Gillham's product CALM). I take it with food.

Nausea – Take prescription drugs to stop throwing up. I also ate applesauce or drank apple juice to calm the stomach and give me a little sugar.

Gas/farting. Yes it may happen often. Just deal with it.

MOVING AND RESTING

WALK – even if it is just around the house – every day. You will yawn a lot as you wake up from the sleepiness of the drugs and that stuck energy releases so you can confront the environment.

Stay in communication with your body. If it's too much to sit up on the first few days after surgery or chemo, lie down.

Keep feet elevated if they start swelling and eat diuretic foods: watermelon, asparagus, and cranberry juice.

Get ear plugs and an eye shade, or pull your stocking cap down over your eyes so you can sleep during daylight hours.

SHOPPING LIST

SUPPLIES:

_____ Cotton balls

_____ Band-aids

_____ Alcohol

_____ Alcohol wipes

_____ Paper towels

_____ Paper plates

_____ Kleenex

_____ Plastic garbage bags

_____ Vagisil/Vagicaine

_____ Baby wipes (unscented)

_____ Sanitary pads to keep Vagisil cream from getting on your underwear

_____ Zantac/Prilosec (magnesium ingredient helped bowel movement)

_____ Extra-strength TUMS

_____ Advil (ask your doctor)

_____ Laxative (ask your doctor)

_____ Antibiotic cream

_____ Hair clippers - When hair falls out shave your head with clippers.

_____ Large hand-held mirror

_____ Nail clippers and nail file

_____ Plastic waste basket (next to your bed if you get sick)

_____ Soft toothbrush

_____ Baking soda

_____ Salt (rinse mouth with salt and baking soda)

_____ Olive oil

_____ Funny movies

_____ Beautiful pictures

_____ Great music

FOOD:

_____ Non-spicy food

_____ Water!

_____ Apple or cranberry juice

_____ Applesauce

_____ Yogurt

_____ Foods to flush body: watermelon, asparagus, cranberry juice

_____ Avoid salt! Too much water retention

_____ Fresh fruits and vegetables

_____ Gelatin (helps re-build fingernails)

_____ High-quality liquid or tablet vitamins

CLOTHES:

_____ Loose-fitting, cotton, slip-on pants with pockets

_____ Zip-up tops with pockets for Kleenex. Easy to slip on and off

_____ Slip-on shoes

_____ Caps for warm and cool weather, and sleeping

_____ Pretty wrap-around head scarf

_____ Wigs – make sure they are adjustable – not too tight or hot

MY TREATMENT JOURNAL

Date of Treatment/Appointment:

Time of Treatment:

Type of Treatment:

Location:

Doctor:

Weight: Blood Pressure: Pulse:

Temperature:

Blood test results:

Other test results:

Discussion notes with doctor/specialist:

Follow-up appointment and action:

Wins/Celebrations:

References, Websites, Organizations

TREATMENT:

Learning about cancer, research, resources, treatment, the American Cancer Society: http://www.cancer.org/

INSPIRATION:

Steve Jobs speech "How to Live Before You Die"
http://www.ted.com/talks/steve_jobs_how_to_live_before_you_die.html

MUSIC:

I Hope You Dance (Lee Ann Womack)
http://www.youtube.com/watch?v=RV-Z1YwaOiw

I Believe I Can Fly (R. Kelly)
http://www.youtube.com/watch?v=QTahrYXCChI

Every Day is Mine (Eric Meyersfield)
http://www.reverbnation.com/ericmeyersfield

Rise (Michael Duff) http://www.michaelduff.com/

Tomorrow Will Come (Wil Seabrook) http://wilseabrook.com/

FINANCES:

Bankruptcy books from Nolo Press: http://www.nolo.com/products/

U.S. Dept of Justice approved credit counseling agencies:
http://www.justice.gov/ust/eo/bapcpa/ccde/

BODY:

Peter Gillham's vitamins website: http://www.vites.com/

Dr. Stephen Price's vitamins website:
http://drpricesvitamins.com/other-vitamins.html

CHARITIES:

National Breast Cancer Foundation:
http://www.nationalbreastcancer.org

Susan G. Komen for the Cure: http://ww5.komen.org

Avon Foundation for Women: http://www.avonfoundation.org

Cancer Care: http://cancercare.org

Look Good…Feel Better: http://lookgoodfeelbetter.org

Charity Watch: http://www.charitywatch.org/toprated.html

Post Script – I Will: Thank You

"Who will build the fire?"

"I will."

THANK YOU:

To Suzy, for giving me the healing diary to make notes on this journey. PS: Suzy is an artist who makes beautiful jewelry and draws lovely pictures and dances with joy, but won't admit she has all that artistic talent. But I will keep telling her until she does.

To Sue, for your friendship, support, and encouragement for my work as a writer. Every day, a new release!

To Carlo, who shoved me into this project after repeatedly asking me, "Where's the book?" And for his undying friendship throughout our time together. He talks tough. But he's a teddy bear. Don't tell anybody.

To my 'navigators' Nery and Johana, and all the hospital staff, doctors and nurses at Olive View Medical Center in Sylmar, California. Keep patchin' these bodies up. We'll keep 'em movin' forward.

To Drs. Wortham and Shields at the Optimum Wellness Group. Thank you for pointing me in the right direction early on. You are spiritual physicians, handling body and soul.

To the Breast and Cervical Cancer Treatment Program, ORSA and Medi-Cal. If anyone tries to cancel these lifesavers, call your elected representative!

To the charities and all who give to them: American Cancer Society, Avon Cares for Life, the Revlon/UCLA Breast Center, and Cancer Care.

To my loving family, who has supported me spiritually, emotionally, and financially, through this adventure. I may be far away, but never far away.

To the public and especially the staff at my church. Your rock-solid ethics, unwavering intention, and dedication to freeing us all as spiritual beings are the highest calling anyone can aspire to. I am proud to call you my friends.

To YOU, the reader of this book. Thank you for purchasing it and helping yourself and others live a healthier life.

May you flourish and prosper.

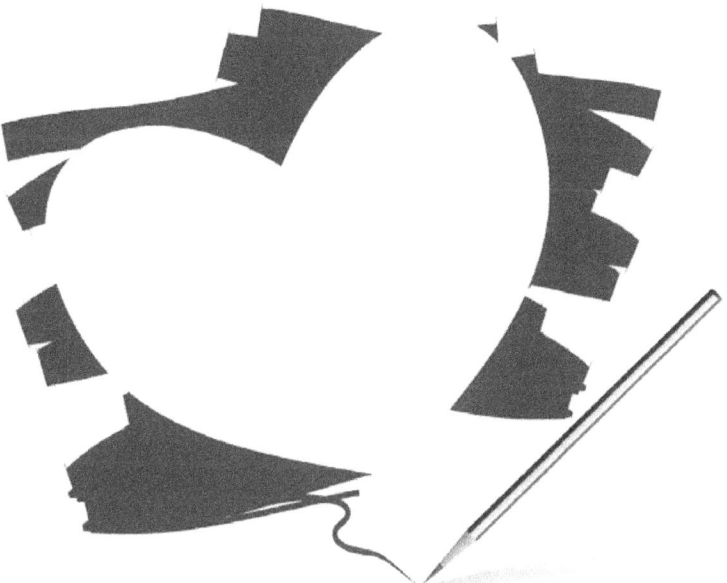

www.ingramcontent.com/pod-product-compliance
Lightning Source LLC
Chambersburg PA
CBHW070201290526